CPR for Caregivers

To Cheryl
With Care
[signature]

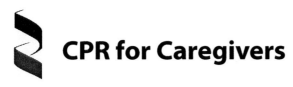

CPR for Caregivers

Connect, **P**roject, and **R**eflect through
Mind, Body, and Spirit

written by
  Grant Watkins

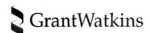 GrantWatkins

Tasora

Printed in the United States of America on acid-free paper.

ISBN 978-1-934690-01-7

Cover design by Kyle G. Hunter
Interior design by Rachel Holscher
Design, typesetting, and printing by BookMobile
Cover photo by Matt Halley

To order additional copies of this book, please go to:
www.itascabooks.com

To Mom and Dad,

for teaching me what it means to be human.

Contents

Author's Note ix
Acknowledgments xi

Introduction 1
How to Connect 15
Connecting with Your Mind 17
Connecting with Your Body 22
Connecting with Your Spirit 28
How to Project 35
Projecting with Your Mind 36
Projecting with Your Body 41
Projecting with Your Spirit 44
How to Reflect 49
Reflecting with Your Mind 51
Reflecting with Your Body 58
Reflecting with Your Spirit 65

Conclusion 71
About the Author 75

Author's Note

It is with great honor that I have been able to serve our most vulnerable and learn from the people who loved them the most.

To respect the privacy of the families and individuals described in this book, the names and events described in *CPR for Caregivers* have been changed.

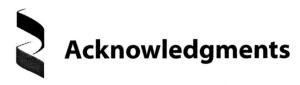 # Acknowledgments

First, I would like to thank Pat Samples, my editor and writing mentor. My thanks also go to Matt Halley for his professional and personal support and for encouraging me to show up when I didn't think I could.

I would also like to thank my mother, Kitsy Watkins Boyd, mother in spirit Elaine Cohen, and family members Alton, Daphne, Ginger, Robert, Shane, Zach, and Tori.

Thanks to the friends and families who have encouraged me in life: Jim Foltz, Young Bebus, Brent Longtin, Deb Sakry-Lande, Wally Kammiere, Wanda Anstett, Betty Marcus-Randle, Scott Hippert, the families of Joe and Juanita Le Desma, John and Q Duke, Charles and Barbara Horak, and Bob and Betty Berryhill.

Introduction

"Your dad can't see," I recall my mom telling me in a quivering voice sometime after my seventeenth birthday. She stood in front of the stove, stirring a pot of Malt-o-Meal.

"What do you mean, he can't see?" I exclaimed.

Mom remained silent, took a deep breath, and held back her tears as she poured the hot cereal into separate bowls for me and my sister. "Hurry up and eat, you're running late for school."

I sat down next to Dad, who was already sitting at the kitchen table with his shoulders and head drooping. For the first time I realized that his diabetes was not going to get any better and he was beginning to surrender to its symptoms. It was a turning point not only for him but also for my entire family. There would be no more eye surgeries, and a very long journey had begun. After dad was declared legally blind, his ill health forced him into early retirement. A year later, he was placed on kidney dialysis.

This isn't supposed to happen to a man in his forties, I thought to myself. *Dad is a strong man—a high school football coach and teacher.*

Over the years, my sister Ginger and I assisted Mom as Dad's primary caregivers. We did everything from cooking and cleaning to bathing, dressing, grooming, and toileting. Ginger helped Mom with the daily insulin injections and the changing of Dad's dialysis bags. I would often cut his toenails and give him foot massages, and Ginger and I both helped Mom out by running errands and by taking Dad to his countless doctor appointments.

We all pitched in because we loved Dad and also felt a sense of obligation to care for him. But over time I felt the sacrifice was too much, and I began to feel burnt out. I was angry at Dad for getting sick and angry at God for making him sick. I was angry with my mom for staying with a man who had abused her in the early years of their marriage. I was upset with my older siblings for not being in town to help with our father's care, and most of all I was angry at myself for feeling resentful.

At times it appeared as if things were going to get better for everyone, and then out of nowhere another crisis would come crashing in on us. One night while caring for my father, my mother began to experience severe abdominal cramps. I rushed her to the hospital, and later that evening surgeons worked to repair a ruptured intestine. Her condition was life threatening, and it was unclear if she was going to survive her illness. It was apparent that she would not be able to care for my father until her full recovery.

Dad's care needs were too great for me to handle, so he was also admitted to the hospital. During my sophomore year in college, I spent several weeks going between hospital floors, caring for both Mom and Dad while waiting anxiously for Mom to fully recover. Mom's recovery continued after her release from the hospital, and we were very thankful to have the support of a home health aide to help us care for Dad.

I was amazed to watch as my mother sprang forward from her own illness in order to offer my dad the care he needed. She credits her survival and recovery on friends, family, and the countless nuns at the hospital praying for her, along with an excellent team of Jewish doctors caring for a conservative Southern Baptist woman. Indeed, when we are sick we need the skill of doctors and the prayers of many to recover, but we must also discover our own resiliency to achieve wellness. For my mom, this resiliency came from her ability to know and nurture herself. It was her example that taught me the importance of self-love when caring for others.

So, for more than five years I cared for Dad. During this journey I felt a litany of emotions, including anger, hurt, disbelief, resentment, compassion, grief, and, of course, love. Shortly after my twenty-second birthday, on a Sunday night I came home to discover my mother standing next to my father. The only thing I can recall her saying that night is, "You need to say good-bye to your dad."

As Mom left the room, I fell to my knees and held my father's lifeless body in my arms. I felt the presence of angels in the room bringing Dad's spirit home. In that moment, my resentment disappeared, and I would have done anything to have him back.

Caring for my father at a young age transformed who I would become as an adult and taught me the value of compassion, patience, and understanding. Eventually, this experience led me to work in human services for a nonprofit organization, where I became a manager of independent housing communities for seniors and people who have chronic physical and mental disabilities. The residents I served included people with paraplegia and quadriplegia—some from birth and others as the result of illness or injury. There were also residents with schizophrenia, bipolar disorder, and other mental health challenges. Most of the residents were older people trying to live independently despite their chronological age or various limitations.

Over time I realized that residents who had the support of family and friends appeared to do better then those who did not. This support from others provided a sense of belonging and nurtured their self-worth. Residents who didn't have the support of family and friends were more likely to feel depressed and would often isolate themselves from the rest of the community. Some of these residents had pushed their family and friends away when they became ill; others simply exhausted the people who were caring for them, causing them not to come back.

As I observed the behavior of many residents and their caregivers, I was surprised to discover that sometimes good caregivers are regarded as bad caregivers in spite of their best intentions. I also noticed that when caregivers begin feeling as if they're bad despite all the good they're doing, they're at risk for burning out and withdrawing from the ones they love and serve. I thought back to my mother's commitment to care for my father (and also her parents) while supporting a family. I realized how much self-care she needed to keep feeling good about herself and to avoid burnout. Over time I came to see that self-care, which I call CPR, is essential for all caregivers to avoid burnout.

 ## What Is Caregiver Burnout?

Burnout is a feeling of disconnection from the people you care about. You also lose connection with your own mind, body, and spirit. You may even lose the desire to be of service to the people in your care. Burnout can be prevented if you learn the principles of CPR for Caregivers.

 ## Finding the Connection

One day I overheard one of my residents tell another resident that her daughter never came to visit and that when she did come, she didn't do anything to help her out. I was astonished to hear this because I knew differently. In fact, when I thought back to the previous week, I remembered seeing the woman's daughter coming almost every day after work to check on her mother. Also, since I was the person who collected the monthly rent check, I was aware that the daughter paid her mother's rent. It was written from the daughter's checking account. In addition to what the daughter contributed in time and money, the resident's grandchildren made several trips to the building each week to provide food, to visit with her, and to clean her apartment.

Apparently, the elderly woman was in the beginning stages of Alzheimer's and truly didn't know who was or wasn't in her life. Nonetheless, her daughter chose to dismiss the hurtful things her mother was saying to her directly and to other residents in the building.

No matter how unpleasant her mother was to her, the daughter continued to show up. As I watched her, it was apparent that she came not out of guilt but out of love for herself and her mother. She was effective in caring for her mother because she did not allow her mother's poor behavior to affect how she cared for her. She connected to herself by setting her own realistic expectations of what was or was not possible.

I was reminded of how my mom would also stay connected with herself by controlling how she felt internally despite what might be happening externally. Mom knew that she could not control everything, but she appeared to control her own attitude and beliefs, taking responsibility for the way she was to care for Dad regardless of the behavior or opinions of others.

The resident's daughter and my mother had one primary quality in common: the ability to inwardly communicate with—stay connected with—themselves. They communicated with confidence and remained calm during a crisis. This inner communication and connection renewed them and also drew in other people to support their caregiving. Their attentive and nurturing caregiving was not dependent upon being valued by the ones they were caring for or by anyone else. Rather, it was based upon their ability to connect with their own mind, body and spirit.

Once they connected to themselves they were able to project a sense of confidence that attracted others to them. Their ability to project a positive sense of self-worth came from their inner reflections. It's easy to care for others when you feel valued and appreciated by them, but much more difficult when you don't feel that sense of appreciation. When you connect internally with your mind, body, and spirit, you'll find the strength inside yourself to meet the external challenges that you face in caring for others.

Know Yourself

You may be wondering, "Why all this talk about *me* as the caregiver? I want to learn to be more effective at taking care of *others*, not *myself*." You're not alone. In fact, most caregivers are more comfortable focusing on the care of others than on nurturing themselves. However, the real secret to a satisfying caregiving experience is understanding that in order to be an effective caregiver, you must first know yourself and you must use that knowledge to nurture yourself. By knowing and nurturing yourself, you will have the energy and desire to nurture others.

Climbing the Spiral Staircase

In order to describe CPR for caregivers, I like to use the metaphor of climbing a spiral staircase. At times when ascending these coil-shaped stairs, you may feel that you're walking in circles. You climb and climb, but it seems like you have accomplished very little.

Caregivers find themselves at different places on the staircase, and no two places are ever the same. Today you might be at one place and tomorrow just one tiny step further. Each step forward, whether tiny or huge, gives you new insights about life and yourself that you weren't able to see from the steps below. Each step brings you perspectives that will help strengthen your mind, body, and spirit.

Now imagine the circular handrail that leads you up these steps. This spiral guide represents your life experiences. As you climb the steps, you are encircled by the array of your experiences, such as a conversation in the elevator, a promotion at work, the birth of a child, or the death of a parent. Some of these experiences may seem insignificant; others may alter your life dramatically. These experiences wind you through the spiral stairs of life. When climbing the steps you'll often find these experiences difficult and painful. Yet these difficult experiences provide the *only* path to growth. Each difficulty you meet along the way is a gift that is telling you it's time to connect, project, and reflect again.

Climbing the steps can be challenging and exhausting if you're unaware of how to care for yourself in the process. CPR is a tool for you to use while climbing each step. It will energize you on your journey up the spiral and will help you avoid caregiver burnout.

At the top of the staircase you'll be able to see your life experience in its entirety. You'll discover a sense of truth, inner peace, and wisdom you didn't have before the journey began.

Once you start the climb, you can no longer step back or climb down the stairwell. You only have the present moment—the step you're on and the steps that are in front of you. Each step on your stairwell is taking you to a higher mind-set or consciousness. Although you may think you're stepping backward, you're not, because at each new step you have the experiences of the past that have taught you new skills or given you new insights.

The spiral staircase is a metaphor for the journey of your caregiving experience. Your mind, body, and spirit all need CPR support as you make the challenging climb up this staircase.

What Is CPR for Caregivers?

Everyone knows what CPR in the medical world is—cardiopulmonary resuscitation. Chances are, you've taken a CPR class. You may even have used the technique to save someone's life. But now it's time to learn about another kind of CPR, one you can use to help revive yourself.

CPR for caregivers is a set of principles for healthy communication. By communicating with yourself and with others in a healthy manner, you can avoid burnout and gain energy to care for a loved one who needs you.

Caregiver communication is based on three simple principles: Connect, Project, and Reflect (CPR).

Connect

Giving effective care depends on establishing a mutual bond with the person for whom you're caring. This bond is built on trust, acceptance, and respect. The necessary foundation for developing this bond is connecting with *yourself.*

Project

The way you communicate with others (what you *project*), whether verbally or nonverbally, can enhance or obstruct the connection. Be aware of what you project so that the connection remains strong.

Reflect

Your positive or negative thoughts (reflections) determine how you project to others. Learn to keep your reflections positive.

By using these principles, you will have the energy to become your own renewable resource. Having an increased level of energy will allow you to respond appropriately to the daily decisions you have to make for your loved one. Having an abundance of positive energy will also attract the right people into your life who will support you in caring for yourself and your loved one.

Each of us has many circles of support—family members, friends, doctors, nurses, social workers, and others. As the trust in these relationships grows, we form strong bonds that hold us together in the toughest of times.

Making connections is critical for every caregiver, but before you can make a strong connection on the outside, you have to make a connection on the inside. You need to be connected to your mind, body, and spirit. Connect with your mind by giving it opportunities to be pleasantly stimulated and refreshed. Make a connection with your body by getting exercise, good nutrition, and adequate sleep. Find ways to make a connection, including developing a relationship with your Higher Power. These are just some of the ways to connect with your mind, body, and spirit that I'll share with you in this book.

Once you've connected with yourself, you're ready to use the tools of projection and reflection to connect with others.

Remember the last movie you went to? On the screen were images that invoked your emotions. What you saw on the screen made you feel good or bad. At the back of the room was a projector that was casting these images onto the screen, stirring up your emotions. Your life is much the same as a movie. The way you express yourself to others is your screen, and what you reflect upon most is sent through the projector and becomes an image on the screen. You can use your screen to empower people and help heal them, or you can use your screen to abuse and suppress others.

As a caregiver, you want to convey self-confidence to those in your care and to others around you. Among the ways you can project this self-confidence are through smiling, making eye contact, showing enthusiasm, and listening attentively. These verbal and nonverbal projections of yourself represent how you see yourself and what you reflect on.

What you reflect upon most is what you're going to project to others, either consciously or unconsciously. You have the power to control both negative and positive thoughts. You can learn to take charge of your thoughts, rather than let them control you. In particular, people like people who like themselves, so thinking positively about yourself will make it easier for people to be around you and to give you support.

As you ascend the caregiving "staircase," good communication results from the way you connect, project, and reflect. Take time to put Caregiver CPR into action, and begin to experience the joy in caregiving.

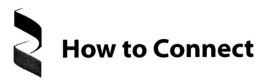

How to Connect

Caregiver burnout is the main barrier to your connecting with others and with yourself. This state of disconnection may show up as depression, anxiety, stress, or fatigue. Several of these symptoms may even show up at the same time. Any of them can affect how you care for others and yourself. To prevent or to respond to these symptoms, self-care is essential for you, especially if you're coping with your own physical and mental health issues while also caring for others. Only through self-care can you reconnect with yourself and find satisfaction again in caregiving.

Remember the spiral staircase representing the journey of the caregiver? Perhaps the hardest part of climbing the steps is having the willingness to take the steps that will connect you to yourself. As a caregiver, you face many demands, and you may feel guilty when you take time out for yourself. Self-care is an important step in connecting with others. When you're connected to yourself, you then have the energy to connect with others. Every time you connect with someone, you're creating a new experience based on what you project and how you reflect. As you choose to connect, project, and reflect in healthy ways, you create experiences that will help you work your way up the staircase. These experiences become the basis for relationships that will help you grow as a person and as a caregiver.

This is not to say that a connection to others always feels good. Not all relationships will be mutually nurturing. In fact, some of your caregiving relationships may be extremely difficult. However, they're just as important as your mutually nurturing relationships because they can help you grow emotionally and spiritually as long as you maintain your commitment to connection.

Every step you take will create an experience with family members, friends, professional helpers, and others. The bonds of trust you develop with these people over time will strengthen you and support you in taking the next step up. These relationships can help hold you together in the toughest of times. Making connections is critical for every caregiver, but before you can make a strong connection on the outside, you have to make a connection on the inside.

Start with self-care. In order to connect to others, you must connect with yourself first. You'll be amazed at the people you'll attract into your life when you feel connected to yourself.

Your success as a caregiver begins with connecting with your mind, body, and spirit. When you connect with these three aspects of yourself, they can work together as one, and you become more integrated as a person. In turn, you will have a solid foundation for handling the challenges of caring for yourself and your loved ones.

Connecting with Your Mind

Every day you make decisions that affect your loved one. Having a sharp mind will allow you to make the best possible decisions. It will also help you develop the skills you need to give good care.

You must balance your work with play by giving your mind mental breaks that are both relaxing and energizing. There are many things you can do to exercise your mind and give you mental breaks from the demands of being a caregiver.

Success Story

Matthew and Mary were married for over forty years when Mary was diagnosed with Alzheimer's. Matthew found himself exhausted with the daily task of caring for his wife, but what really worried him was whether he would be able to keep things straight in his own mind. Would he remember to give Mary her medication? How would he keep track of the various doctor appointments? Eventually Matthew and Mary decided to sell their home and move into an independent housing community with services. For Matthew, this decision took a big load off his mind because he knew that help was just a phone call away should his wife need the services of a personal care attendant.

In their new setting, Matthew found a number of new ways to keep his sanity by exercising his mind. He joined in activities at the housing community. Among his favorites were bingo, dominos, and cards. When Matthew felt the need to stay close to Mary, he worked on a daily crossword puzzle inside their apartment.

Mary had many medical needs, and Matthew often felt overwhelmed by the challenges of caring for his wife. Participating in social activities in his community allowed him to take mental breaks from the daily task of caring for Mary. It also helped him maintain his memory.

Paula, the couple's daughter, also helped care for Mary. Paula often felt overwhelmed by the difficulties

of caregiving. She started a book club with some la-
dies from her condominium community. This allowed
her the mental break that she needed in order to help
manage her mother's health care needs.

What You Can Do

It's okay for you to take a mental break from caregiving.
In fact, you'll find it beneficial, and so will your loved one.
If you think you don't have time to take a break, think
again. Just like our bodies need rest, so do our minds.
Giving your mind a break allows you to come back to
your caregiving responsibilities with a sense of mental
clarity and renewal.

Having mental clarity allows you to be more objective
when handling the daily decisions of caregiving. It also
helps reduce the amount of frustration that is common
for all caregivers. Unless you take mental breaks, mount-
ing frustration may cause you to burn out, leaving you
with a sense of hopelessness.

You may be thinking that you can't take a mental
break because you're the only one who can care for your
loved one. Try to come up with a list of people who might
be willing to help out, and ask for what you need. You'll
be surprised at how many people want to help if you ask

them. Begin by asking family and friends. You may even want to contact your faith community and ask if there are any members who can give an hour or two a week to help so you can take a break. Or perhaps you belong to other groups that may be willing to provide some volunteer assistance. Paid helpers are also available to come in for a time so you can get away.

Becoming involved in your community is another great way to exercise your mind while also giving you a break from your caretaking responsibilities. Here are some ideas that other caregivers have found helpful:

Connect with socializing

While caring for a loved one, it's easy to isolate yourself from the rest of the world. Take time to stay connected with people in your life and reach out to new friends by socializing with people who share your intellectual and social interests. You may find that many of the people you meet have had similar caregiving experiences.

Connect with part-time work

The right part-time job can give you a needed break from your role of caregiving. It can also help offset some of the financial concerns you might be having.

Connect with learning and hobbies

Below is a list of fun and educational activities that some caregivers have told me they use to connect with their mind. Use this list to help you think of activities that will relax and stimulate you.

- Knitting
- Scrapbooking
- Organizing old photos
- Traveling
- Oil painting
- Music lessons
- Photography
- Writing
- Playing cards
- Taking a class at a local college or university
- Exploring new interests on the Internet

Connect with volunteering

Reaching out in service to others is a way to connect with your mind. Think about organizations, programs, and causes that are meaningful to you. How can you be of service to those groups now? Serving others that are in need can help you become more grateful for the things you have. At the same time, it can give you a mental break and relieve stress in your own life.

The Benefits of Connecting with Your Mind

Remember that the key to being an effective caregiver is knowing how to care for yourself. When you take the time to connect with your mind, you'll experience many rewards, including:

- Better memory
- Renewed energy
- More self-confidence
- Stronger relationships
- Less stress
- Lower blood pressure
- Less worry

Connecting with Your Body

Caregivers burn out when they disconnect from their bodies. Proper nutrition, exercise, and sleep are important for everyone. Caregivers have a tendency to neglect themselves while caring for others, sacrificing their own health in the process.

Success Story

Marie, who works full-time, was looking forward to an early retirement with her husband. Marie received a horrible call one day. Her father had died unexpectedly, and she not only suddenly begins grieving the loss of her father but also caring for her mother.

Money had always been a problem for Marie's parents, and her mother now finds it necessary to sell the family home in order to pay off funeral expenses and keep up with medical bills. Since she's never developed the skills to manage money, she has to rely on Marie for help with handling her finances. At the same time, she's feeling a great deal of grief over the loss of her husband, and she doesn't like the idea of leaving her home. In the midst of all the distress she is feeling, she questions and resents some of the financial decisions Marie is making for her.

Marie feels frustrated with the situation. She knows that her mother has to move or face foreclosure, and she's willing to help take care of her mother's affairs. However, her mother has become extremely combative and often undermines many of the decisions Marie makes. Marie's husband was supportive initially, but he has begun to lose his patience and wants Marie to distance herself from her mother. He's upset that Marie's mother is unappreciative of anything the two of them do to help.

The stress has caused Marie stress in her body. She experiences migraine headaches and feelings of anxiety. Marie has discovered that exercise reduces her overall discomfort. Walking thirty minutes a day several times a week on a nature trail near her home allows her time by herself and has also helped her lose excess weight. Marie loves walking, and it allows her to connect with her body and with nature. She comes back from her walks feeling refreshed and able to think more clearly.

While on the nature trail, Marie has also become very interested in bird-watching. This new hobby has allowed Marie to exercise her mind while exercising her body. If the weather is bad, Marie walks at the local mall to get exercise.

Another thing that aggravates Marie's anxiety is the fact that her younger brother visits his mother a few times a month but is unable or unwilling to provide some of the necessary care for her. Recently, Marie sat down with her siblings and made out a list of her mother's care needs. The list was then divided among all three of Marie's siblings. Marie's younger brother is now held accountable for some of their mother's care plan.

Also, Marie and her husband are working together on a financial plan that would share the financial responsibilities with Marie's siblings.

Having written out a care plan for her mother and having delegated some of the responsibilities to her siblings, Marie has been able to reconnect with her body more easily. Her stress level is down because she does not feel the heavy burden of caring for her mother alone. This has allowed Marie to realize that things don't have to be perfect to work. Since Marie has reconnected with herself, her husband has been more understanding about Marie's desire to help her mother out financially.

What You Can Do

Proper nutrition, sleep, and exercise are critical when connecting with the body. It would be hard to survive without these basics, yet they often are neglected when the care of others is put before the care of ourselves.

Connect with nutrition

In your busy life as a caregiver, it's easy to forget the importance of healthy eating. Avoid the fast-food rut and make healthy snacks when you're on the go. Pick up some fresh fruit, vegetables, and nutrition bars that you can eat when you're too busy to prepare a full meal. This will help you avoid "bingeing" on the empty calories found in most convenience foods.

Connect with sleep

Sleep is essential for the caregiver. Many caregivers suffer from insomnia that may be caused by emotional or physical problems. If you have a hard time sleeping, check with your doctor to explore any underlying cause of your sleep deprivation. Here are some additional ways to help you sleep:

- Bedtime preparation—Watch when and what you eat before you go to sleep. Start the night right by avoiding caffeine and alcohol before bedtime and sticking to a regular bedtime routine.
- Open your eyes—If you're tired but can't fall asleep, try keeping your eyes open. The more you focus on keeping your eyes open, the harder it will be to do so. Before you know it, you'll be sleeping like a baby.
- Sound—Sometimes a constant sound can help you sleep. Try running a white noise machine, a fan, or an air filter system.

Connect with exercise

Exercise can change your mood and reduce stress. Engage in some type of physical activity at least three times a week to energize yourself from the inside out. Here are a few exercise ideas to consider:

- Yoga—Strength and flexibility are only a few benefits of yoga. You will also learn how to stay balanced and to relax.
- Swimming—Take the plunge and treat your whole body to a workout. Swimming can be learned at any age, so jump in and start feeling good again.
- Adult basketball—Who says basketball is only for kids? Contact your YMCA or local gym and ask if they have any amateur teams you can play on.
- Dancing—It's fun and it's great exercise. Find a friend and check out your local community center. Most centers offer beginner classes, and prices are reasonable. Bring your dancing shoes and learn Latin, polka, salsa, line dancing, or swing.
- Self-defense—Learning to defend yourself is important for people of all ages. Classes teach the basics such as how to get out of a hold and how to boost your confidence in a challenging situation.
- Tae Kwon Do—Kick, punch, and strike are only

a few of the things you will learn in Tae Kwon Do. It will also help build discipline, focus, and endurance.

- Community theater—Ever dreamed about being on the big screen? Why not start at your local community theater? Acting is a great way to connect with your body. It will also provide you with the opportunity to meet some of your neighbors, have fun, and expand your creativity—a much-needed resource for caregivers!

The Benefits of Connecting with Your Body

- More resiliency
- Fewer illnesses
- Better health
- Greater vitality
- More self-confidence
- Less stress

 Connecting with Your Spirit

Caregivers often rely on their mind and body but often fail to nurture their spirit. Your spirit opens the door to connect with others and also connects you with the circle of life. Inside the circle of life you feel connected to the very source that created you.

Your spirit is what gives you hope when you feel hopeless and brings light where there is darkness. You can connect to your spirit in many ways. Some of my favorites include listening to relaxing music, experiencing intentional silence, and enjoying the wonders of nature.

Success Story

Julie and Frank, a retired couple who live on a small fixed income, have been caring for Ethel, Frank's mother, for three years. Julie and Frank feel an obligation to care for Ethel because she is family and they truly care about her, but they are exhausted from frequent travel between their Rhode Island home and Ethel's home in upstate New York. Ethel's physical needs are being met in New York, but she longs for the personal attention of her son. Frank feels guilty about his mother being so far away and makes the five-hour drive to see her several times a month. Julie and Frank have received a number of calls from Ethel's care attendant requesting that they come immediately to help Ethel with a health care crisis. The couple has asked Ethel to move closer to them, but she has refused. Julie and Frank can't leave their local community because they're also caring for their grandchildren who live nearby.

Both Julie and Frank find strength from their faith. Julie prays every day for the well-being of her mother-in-law and for the protection of their family. Members of their faith community are also supportive of Julie and Frank. When Frank has to make the drive to New York by himself and spend a few days away from home, members of their congregation bring food over for Julie or invite her out to eat. They also pray for the couple and take turns making weekly visits to their home, giving Julie and Frank opportunities to talk over their concerns with understanding people.

The pastor of their church has also provided Frank and Julie spiritual guidance. He listens to them and validates them. He reminds them that Ethel's care is in the hands of their Higher Power, and he supports their decision to stay close to their grandchildren.

Frank has found a way to eliminate some of the guilt that he feels by volunteering at his church, making home visits to other elders in their town. Sometimes he provides transportation to medical appointments or drives someone to the grocery store. Frank believes that he is connecting to his spirit by serving others. While he can't be in New York all the time to assist his mother, he feels good about providing loving support to older adults close to home.

What You Can Do

Connect with your Higher Power

Your Higher Power (however you define that for yourself) can be your main source of strength and carry you through difficult times. For some people, connecting with a Higher Power is not easy because they've had negative experiences with religion and may have even suffered spiritual abuse within their faith-based communities. If you don't feel at home with the religion of your past or have unresolved anger towards your Higher Power, consider looking for a new religious or spiritual home with a belief system that supports and affirms you for who you are.

Connect with music

My favorite way to connect to my spirit is through music. Let your spirit dance to the beat of a drum or the sound of a beautiful tune. Instrumental music works best for me. You can also try singing, chanting, or even humming to help you connect with your spirit.

Connecting with nature

Take a walk outside and discover something new. Nature has a way of connecting us to our spirit. Take a look at all of life's most precious creatures. Notice what the atmosphere is doing. Feel the wind, feel the rain, let the sunshine beat down on your skin, and connect yourself with nature.

Connecting with silence

All the wisdom you need is within you, and you can tap into this wisdom when you surrender to silence in a time of reflection by yourself. Your life experience will give you the answers if you take time to listen. Be open to what you hear and follow your intuition.

The Benefits of Connecting with Your Spirit

- An overall sense of peace
- Deep states of relaxation
- Less stress
- Significant personal insight
- Sense of wholeness

Concluding Thoughts on Connecting

Connecting with your mind, body, and spirit forms a foundation that renews you and allows you to care for yourself and others. When you feel a strong connection to yourself, you can more easily connect with others.

Having this strong foundation also allows you to be consciously aware of how you communicate with yourself and others. Good communication begins with taking responsibility for the decisions you make about taking care of yourself.

Connecting to your mind allows you the freedom to choose how you'll spend your time in caring for yourself or others. By taking mental breaks when necessary and truly enjoying your life when you are not a caregiver, you'll have the ability to create personal boundaries that will support you in your caregiving role.

Connecting with your body through proper nutrition, exercise, and sleep provides your body with the energy, strength, and rest you need to care for others. It also helps to sustain your health and well-being so that you can take care of your own needs.

Connecting with your spirit allows you to experience inner peace. You may find that connection from being part of a faith-based community that affirms you, through making or listening to music, or by spending time in nature. Everyone's spiritual needs are different, so do what works for you, not what you think others want you to do.

Once you've spent time connecting with yourself, you can start connecting with others. You'll be successful in connecting with others by how you project and reflect. Remember that the support of others strengthens you as you ascend those stairs.

How to Project

Can you think of a time when the person you're caring for failed to appreciate all you've been doing for him or her? You may have even been treated with disrespect despite your efforts to love and serve unconditionally.

Many caregivers feel guilt and uneasiness over circumstances they have no power to control, yet these same circumstances often control them and keep them from making plans in their own life. They may have contributed emotionally, physically, and financially to the person they care for, yet that person speaks ill of them behind their back or directly to them. They may find themselves being judged by other members of their family who question their ability to provide the appropriate care for their loved one. They may experience an array of such hurtful attitudes and behaviors being *projected* by others.

If you've had this type of experience, your sense of self-worth may have taken a hit, and you may not feel very willing to connect to others. You may find yourself becoming depressed and isolated or snapping at others for no apparent reason. It's easy to get caught up in projecting negatively onto others the very attitudes and behaviors that others have projected onto you.

 Projecting with Your Mind

Although you can't control how others are going to receive or perceive you, you do have control over how you receive and perceive their negativity. You can choose your own attitudes and behavior, which in turn you'll project back to them and others.

When I was managing a building serving people with chronic physical and mental disabilities, one resident, who was paraplegic since birth, would cuss and spit at me. For a month I tried to build a positive relationship with him by discussing common events in the community and our common interests. No matter what I said or did, he rejected my kindness. Finally, one day I asked him why he disliked me so much. His eyes filled with tears, and then he said, "Because you can walk and I can't."

This man taught me that caregivers who take the behaviors of others personally place themselves at high risk of burning out. Sometimes what others project onto us has nothing to do with the way we're treating them but is based upon what they reflect on in their own lives. You can't be responsible for how others are going to receive or perceive you, but you *are* accountable for how you connect to yourself and handle what others project to you.

Whether you're projecting consciously or unconsciously, verbally or nonverbally, you have the power to influence others when you project from the way you feel inside. When you act with acceptance, trust, and respect, you nurture enthusiasm in yourself and in others. When the person you're caring for experiences your enthusiasm, he or she feels a sense of hope.

Once you've learned how to positively affect the way others feel about themselves, you have mastered the art of projection. I've spoken to many caregivers who doubt their effectiveness in caring for others because they lack confidence. Some feel this way because, as they grow older, they can't think as fast as they once did or they have problems remembering things.

Projecting positively comes from your heart and into your mind. It has nothing to do with your skills but everything to do with enthusiasm. Sharing your enthusiasm with others is what projecting with your mind is all about. If you use your mind to bring out the best in others, you will soon have the support of others that will help you climb your way to the top of the stairway.

Success Story

Chuck and Stacy have been married for ten years and are raising a six-year-old girl and a five-year-old boy. Chuck was a soldier for a few years and was injured by a roadside bomb while serving in Iraq. The explosion caused Chuck to suffer a traumatic brain injury, which has hampered his ability to communicate with his wife and kids.

Chuck suffers from post-traumatic stress disorder and often drinks alcohol to cope with the mental and physical limitations he now has. His continued heavy drinking could cause permanent damage to his physical body and emotional damage to his marriage. Stacy does not completely understand the complexities of post-traumatic stress disorder, and her lack of knowledge has impacted how she treats her husband.

Stacy expected her husband to recover quickly from the incident and doesn't feel that he is contributing to his own healing. She feels angry over the poor care he is receiving, and she's having a difficult time adjusting to her new life with him. Stacy often loses her temper with Chuck. She snaps at him when he does not comprehend what she's saying.

Stacy's behavior is affecting their kids. They have begun to mimic Stacy's behavior, yelling at their father and losing patience with his slow mobility.

Stacy recently joined a support group that is helping her cope with her loss and her frustrations with Chuck's behavior. She has learned to control her temper and has begun to communicate with her children about the severity of their father's injuries. The group has helped her learn that comparing herself to others only leads to feelings of inadequacy. The family is now learning about Chuck's illness and disabilities in an effort to better serve him. Learning to communicate openly and sharing their wisdom with others has brought the family closer together.

What You Can Do

Project with honesty

Talking about the hard stuff can often minimize worry and concern.

Project with enthusiasm

Your enthusiasm creates positive energy that can be very healing and will attract positive people into your life.

Project with integrity

Doing what you say you're going to do builds trust.

Project with listening

Listening is healing. When you listen without judgment, you're practicing unconditional love.

Project with confidence

Act with caring confidence. People find this behavior attractive and want to be around it.

Project with authenticity

Be yourself, even if you're different from the people around you.

Project with humor

Caring for others is tough work. Finding the humor in it can get you through some very difficult times.

The Benefits of Projecting with Your Mind

- The joy that comes from inspiring others
- Discovery of how this joy is contagious
- Greater emotional intimacy

- Authentic self-expression
- Transformation of the emotional landscape of others

Projecting with Your Body

When you are speaking to others, some of what you say comes through voice and some through body language. If what you're saying doesn't match up with what your body is saying, you'll have a difficult time influencing the people you care about.

Your gestures are an important part of your message. You can use them to your advantage to support the message that is coming from your voice.

Success Story

The best day of Jack's life was the day he and his partner adopted a six-week-old baby boy named Tommy. Jack was well aware that his son was born with physical challenges and would eventually have to undergo traumatic surgeries to repair a cleft palate and issues in his digestive tract. What Jack didn't know was that his son was also autistic and would live out his life being nonverbal.

Tommy's care team included doctors, nurses, social

workers, and personal care attendants. Raising the little boy created many challenges in Jack's relationships, and he soon found himself raising Tommy by himself. Over the years, Tommy and Jack developed a deep, loving bond. Their only way of communicating was through nonverbal physical expressions. Tommy would open his arms when he wanted to be held. When he wanted his independence, Tommy would hold his hands out with his palms facing Jack.

Jack realized early on that physical gestures were the easiest way he could communicate with his young son. Now that Tommy is eight years old, Jack still uses this form of communication to express the profound love he has for his son, and Tommy responds to the gentle touch of his father, especially when he is feeling overstimulated.

When we communicate, we use more than just our voice. Our gestures help us to express ourselves. The people in our care will make judgments based upon what they see in our body.

If what you're saying doesn't match up to your body language, then you may come across as insincere. People may have a hard time trusting you, which may keep you walking in circles and prevent you from climbing up the spiral staircase.

What You Can Do

Project with a smile

Your smile tells the world what's in your heart. It can inspire others to feel good about themselves.

Project with eye contact

The eyes are the doorway to a person's soul and can be a way to express trust. Trust is the cornerstone for building a circle of support as we care for others.

Project with body movement

Your body movement is a reflection of what your mind is thinking. If you're nervous, tense, or feeling insecure, this feeling will be expressed in the way you move your body or perhaps grip your hands and arms. Open your hands and arms wide to express empathy, allowing the one you care for to feel that you understand.

Project with voice

Your voice is the most powerful tool you have to convey a message. You can use your voice to express meaning by speaking loudly or softly, harshly or gently. However you use your voice, remember that your words can help heal or hurt the one you are caring for.

The Benefits of Projecting with Your Body

- Warm, trusting relationships
- Greater sense of confidence
- Creating fond memories
- Connecting to others

 Projecting with Your Spirit

Have you ever met people who had charisma? I'm sure you will agree they were personable, well-liked, and had the ability to influence others in their environment. On TV we witness a person like Oprah Winfrey who can influence large populations in a matter of minutes. People with charisma have learned to project with their spirits.

You can project with your spirit by living your life authentically. Projecting with your spirit means living what you preach. Nobody likes a phony, and people who live authentically are living what they believe.

Many caregivers feel stressed and become burned out because there is a gap between what they think and how they feel. You can lessen this gap by truly living in service to others. If you feel burned out, ask your Higher Power how you can best serve the people you care for. Then listen for the answer. New ideas and thoughts will form, giving you the direction and energy to do what is needed. When you transform your positive thoughts into actions, you inspire others.

Success Story

In 2005, I participated in the Red Ribbon Ride, a charity bike ride that raises money for people who have HIV or AIDS. Participants were required to raise $1,500 and ride their bikes over 300 miles in a four-day span.

Although the bike ride was the most physically and emotionally challenging thing I have ever participated in, it was also one of the most transformational. There were many times during the ride that I wanted to give up, especially on the second and third days. The temperature was in the nineties, and the humidity level was high. After being chased by growling dogs and riding my bike for several hours in the hot sun, I suddenly began to feel immense pain in my calves and ankles.

The terrain had changed from flat farmland to a steep uphill climb. As far as the eye could see, it was only uphill, and I didn't think I was going to make it. The pain was very strong, and my thoughts kept telling me to quit. But I also knew that I couldn't quit, that I needed to push myself hard. I prayed, I cried, and at times I cursed the hill as I looked up and saw the long stretch ahead of me. Finally, I came to the realization that the hill was too tough for me to pedal up, and my spirit was ready to give up.

My bike was coming to a slow crawl when an elderly woman zoomed past me on her bike. She yelled out, "One pedal at a time. Don't think about the hill. Just think about the next pedal." Umm, one pedal at a time. When I looked up again, the woman was at the top of the hill taking a break. She had done it, and I was determined to do it, too. I stopped looking at what was ahead of me and started to focus on one pedal at a time. Before I knew it, I was at the top of the hill, but the elderly woman was not there. She had already begun her journey back to our bike camp.

I realized that the woman on the bike thought well of herself. She liked who she was. Her spirit projected these positive feelings and inspired me to keep on biking. We can inspire others by how we project ourselves.

What You Can Do
Project with love

When you love yourself unconditionally, you can love others unconditionally. Allow yourself to be who you are and others to be who they are.

Project with kindness

When you are kind to others, they have a desire to help you climb upward. Kindness is love in action.

Project with forgiveness

When you forgive others, you're setting yourself free from the pain of the past. When you're willing to forgive others, people will be more willing to forgive you.

The Benefits of Projecting with Your Spirit

- Peace of mind
- Connection to your Higher Power
- Trust in your intuition
- Inspiring others around you

 # Concluding Thoughts on Projecting

The preceding chapter introduced you to the importance of connecting with yourself so that you can connect with others. This chapter has examined projection, the second dimension of CPR that helps you connect with others and climb to the next step on the staircase.

Projecting with your mind allows you to express the

positive virtues in which you believe. These virtues inspire others and help to form a sense of trust and authenticity between you and the care receiver. Projecting with your body physically engages those for whom you're caring. How you appear to them or the way your touch assures them can be just as important as what you say to them. Projecting with your spirit gives others a sense of confidence and comfort.

Projection is a product of your thoughts. What you reflect upon, you project. Like you, others project reflections of their own thoughts. The person in your care most likely doesn't feel well physically, emotionally, or spiritually and as a result may project his or her pain to you. Be mindful of this dynamic, and try your best to avoid taking these negative behaviors personally.

The care you're providing is hard work. Some days, taking one step on the staircase requires all your energy. But with each step, remember that you *are* making progress.

How to Reflect

Reflection consists of the positive and negative thoughts that determine how you project to others. What you reflect upon most is what you are going to project to others, either consciously or unconsciously. Successful caregivers learn to control what they reflect on and therefore have control over what they project to others. This allows them to connect with or disconnect from the ones they are caring for or the people in their support circle.

What you reflect on comes from your beliefs about yourself and the world. These beliefs come from what you have learned and experienced since the time you were born.

While managing a senior living building, I met a wonderful lady in her eighties who struggled with poor health but always had a smile on her face and was genuinely happy. Her happiness was contagious, and all the other residents wanted to be around her. Early one morning, as she passed me in the hall, I asked her, "Why are you so happy?" She replied with a smile, "I had a wonderful childhood."

While not all of us had that kind of childhood, fortunately our self-image is constantly shifting based on what we choose to reflect upon and by the new experiences we create with the people in our life. When we reflect in the present moment, our mind, body, and spirit are in harmony. You bring yourself to the present moment by becoming aware of your breathing and conscious of your senses. Pay attention to what you see, hear, taste, smell, or feel. I use this process of being aware of my breath and my senses regularly to check on my thoughts: am I reflecting on what is happening to me in the present moment or on something that has happened to me in the past?

So much of our pain and suffering comes from living in the past or fearing the future. We have no control over the past or the future, but we do have control over the present moment. Only in the present moment can we influence others and have an impact on the future.

How you reflect is the foundation of what you will project and ultimately how you will connect with others. When you become conscious of this cycle of reflecting, projecting, and connecting, you gain increased control over your life.

Reflecting with Your Mind

Many caregivers don't realize that what they reflect on controls their feelings and that negative reflections can cause caregiver burnout. You can take charge of what you reflect on by becoming the observer of the message you hear inside your mind.

Learn to identify yourself as separate from your mind. Allow yourself to observe every thought and then take action to turn negative thoughts into positive ones. Your thoughts will certainly affect how you feel about yourself and others. How you feel inside is an indicator of what you're reflecting on. Change your thoughts and you'll see how fast the uncomfortable feelings go away.

For example, if you're feeling lonely, angry, or afraid, acknowledge the feeling and then ask yourself what you were reflecting on before you started to feel these things. Many caregivers have feelings that are completely un-warranted. They're afraid that if they go out for a night of fun, something might happen to their loved one. This type of fear-based reflection can cause caregiver burnout.

The person you are caring for needs the positive you, not your negative thoughts. If you notice that you are reacting to the person you're caring for with negative thoughts, then take a moment to acknowledge the impact that caring for this person is having on you emotionally, physically, or spiritually. You may be surprised to find out how much your thoughts control your mood and actions. When you acknowledge the negative emotions you're having, you release the negative energy of these emotions. Then you can take steps to renew yourself and become a better caregiver. Only you can change what you're reflecting on.

For example, imagine taking time off from your caregiving duties to go out for a night of fun. If necessary, you could call on one of the many people who are qualified to care for your loved one so you can care for yourself. When imagining taking this time away to have fun, one of your first thoughts might be, "How can you go out and have fun when your husband is home sick?" or "How could you live with yourself if something happens to your wife while you're out tonight?"

These thoughts may come to mind because you've heard such comments from others. People who speak in judgmental terms like this fail to recognize that your health and well-being depend on your taking time out for yourself. When you take care of yourself, you're in a much better position to be an effective caregiver.

Anytime you recognize that you hear one of these

overly cautious, judgmental voices in your mind, write down what it's saying, and restate the message in a way that helps you reflect positively. For example, "I need this night off for me so that I can better serve my husband during the week." Or, "If something does happen to my wife tonight, it's not because I choose to take care of myself."

Are your thoughts preventing you from living in the present moment? If so, then you have let your mind have power over you. By simply observing your thoughts and redirecting them, you can regain your power to care for yourself and your loved one.

Success Story

Duane and Marti have raised three kids. Their oldest two children successfully completed college and graduated with honors. When their youngest son dropped out of college, they were disappointed but knew that college was not for everyone and refrained from judging his decision. They sat down with their son, hoping to help him find a new career path. When they met with their son, they noticed that he appeared withdrawn and aloof.

The following day their young son called his parents and told them that he had been hearing voices. At first Duane and Marti thought he was joking, but with the help of a therapist they realized that their son had schizophrenia. Marti's uncle had been diagnosed with schizophrenia, and she always worried that one of her children would suffer from the same mental illness.

Marti felt responsible for the family genetics that caused her son's schizophrenia. She began to isolate herself because she was ashamed of having this illness in the family. At the same time, many of Marti's friends didn't know how to deal with the stigma of mental illness, so they stopped including Duane and Marti in their social activities. Duane and Marti started to feel like social outcasts, which affected their sense of self-worth and their ability to offer their son the best care possible. Because they felt paralyzed by the shame of having a mentally ill son, they were reluctant to get help. Over time and with the help of counseling, Duane and Marti began to educate themselves about mental illness and eventually stopped feeling guilty about their son's condition. Instead of putting their attention on blaming family genetics for the illness, they began to advocate for people who suffer from mental illness, allowing them to gain power over their lives. Rather than allowing the social stigma associated with mental illness to control their thoughts and feelings, they changed how they viewed

mental illness and are now working to help people who
have mental illness and their caregivers.

The Rules of Self-Esteem

Your thoughts control how you feel. If you want to feel
differently, you need to reflect differently. Turn negative
thoughts into positive thoughts easily by playing a game
that I call "Reflect."

Everyone knows the rules whether they are conscious
of them or not. People who connect in a healthy way with
each other have one thing in common—self-esteem. Self-
esteem is the cornerstone for caregiving. Healthy self-
esteem empowers your independence and gives you the
energy and strength to care for others.

How you reflect can boost your self-esteem. Just play
the game of Reflect by following these simple guidelines:

- Rule #1: Become the observer of what you are reflecting on.
- Rule #2: Notice that what you reflect on deter-
  mines how you feel and that how you feel renews
  you or drains you.
- Rule #3: Control how you feel by changing what
  you reflect on.

Only you can control what you're going to reflect on. Take action today so that you can start enjoying higher self-esteem and more joy in caregiving.

What You Can Do

Reflect with compassion

Self-compassion is taking some of the same love you give to others and giving it to yourself. Self-compassion is a great antidote to self-pity.

Reflect with truth

Check your thoughts for accuracy. We can easily create a lot of "drama" from making assumptions, judgments, or interpretations based on fears or past hurts. Keep your eye on the essential goodness and truth in every situation that will inspire your best.

Reflect with forgiveness

Forgiveness transforms negative thoughts into positive thoughts. Is there someone or something you need to forgive? Start with forgiving yourself.

Reflect with visualization

Visualize yourself as strong and capable of handling anything that comes your way. Remember, we attract what we most think about.

Reflect with a journal

Keep a journal with you to record and change your thoughts. When you notice that you're having upsetting feelings, take a minute to notice the thought(s) that led to you feeling that way. Write the negative thought in your journal. Below that thought, reframe the idea in a positive way. Here are some examples.

Negative thought:

> *I'm afraid that no one else can care for my husband like I do.*

Reframe into a positive thought:

> *Although I love my husband, there are many people who can care for him so that I can take a break from caregiving.*

Negative thought:

> *Why do I always screw things up? I'm not cut out to be a caregiver.*

Reframe into a positive thought:

> *Sometimes my expectations are too high. It's OK for me not to expect so much out of myself. I will do the best that I can, and that's good enough.*

The Benefits of Reflecting with Your Mind

- Clear mind and relaxed body
- Release of guilt, stress, anxiety, and fear
- Control over how you feel and what you do
- Happy emotions and better caregiving

 Reflecting with Your Body

Learn to use your body as a source of information. If you feel tired, perhaps it's time for you to slow down. If you're feeling anxious, do a reality check with your thoughts, or check out the amount of caffeine you're pouring into your body. The aches and pains you're feeling inside your body can sometimes be symptomatic of what you're thinking, eating, or drinking, but they can also be symptomatic of an underlying medical issue. Your doctor can advise you if your aches and pains are related to a serious medical issue. If they're not, give some attention to what you've been thinking, eating, or drinking. You might need to change one of these so that you can feel more comfortable.

Your body will tell you how it feels about what you eat, drink, or think. Take time out to reflect with your body. Does your body feel anxious? That's probably a sign that you're thinking scary thoughts. Check out those thoughts and make some adjustments. Does your body feel tense? That might be a clue that you're judging something or have unrealistic expectations. Again, adjusting what you reflect on can improve how you feel.

Also become conscious of your senses, and listen to what they're telling you. Your senses each have a purpose, and each sense will help you navigate life. Paying attention to your senses helps you live in the present moment.

When you have negative feelings in your body, check in with your senses. What do you see? What do you feel? What do you hear? What can you taste or smell? What are your senses *experiencing in this moment*? Sometimes negative thoughts come to mind when sensory experiences remind us of unpleasant past experiences. But those past experiences have nothing to do with what is really happening now. Give your attention to what you're sensing *now*. When you become conscious of your senses, you're able to distinguish what is truly going on from what you're recalling from the past and even from what you're imagining or anticipating in the future.

Success Story

Jean and John have been married for more than thirty years. When John started having problems with his eyesight last year, Jean insisted that he stop driving. John refused, because to him that meant giving up his independence.

John was tired of hearing his wife nag him about giving up driving, so he agreed to give up driving at night but not during the day. John and Jean were heading into town one afternoon when a storm hit their small rural town. The county road they were on was under construction, and in the intensity of the thunderstorm, John lost control of their station wagon, causing a serious car accident. A pedestrian was injured. Neither Jean nor John was injured in the accident, but Jean began to experience anger over the accident, which manifested in physical pain.

Several people involved in the accident filed suit against Jean and John, and the lawsuits took an emotional and financial toll on both of them. Not long after the accident, they sold their home and moved into an assisted living community where they could get services that would enable them to live independently as they grew older. Despite the beautiful surroundings they were living in, Jean was unable to forgive John for the accident.

When the assisted living community provided outings for the residents, Jean would panic any time they passed road construction. The roar of the tractors and the smell of tar were sensory reminders of what she experienced at the time of the accident. She felt like she was back at the scene of the accident again and experienced a great deal of anxiety. Sometimes Jean would even get angry at John if she looked outside and saw a car that was similar to the one they were driving when they had their accident. It was as though her senses were in overdrive.

With the help of a social worker at the assisted living community, Jean learned to pay attention to her senses, and she can now identify the cause of many of the emotional reactions she has. Awareness of her senses has allowed Jean to check in with herself before getting upset with John. Now that Jean is aware of her senses, she has the power to control how she responds in caring for John instead of her senses controlling her and causing her to burn out.

Over time Jean forgave John for the accident. Eventually, the aches and pains in her body went away. Now when Jean feels physical pain, she listens to what her body is reflecting and sensing. If her senses are recalling the past, she then chooses to focus on different thoughts.

Remember, we experience the world around us

through our senses. Make sure what you are sensing is real and not reflective of a past experience. You can't always control what you are going to see, hear, taste, smell, or feel, but you do have control over how you're going to respond to it.

What You Can Do

Reflect with seeing

For many people, sight is the most important sense they have. The things that you see can make you feel badly and lead to burnout. Seeing people you care about get ill or die can reinforce a sense of helplessness, especially if you have experienced feeling helpless in your past or you're worried about the future. If what you're seeing is starting to burn you out, take a look at something that inspires you in the present. A child laughing or a cat chasing its tail always brings a smile to my face.

Reflect with hearing

The associations you make with certain sounds and noises can have a powerful effect on your mood. When you feel like you're burning out, become conscious of what you hear. Notice whether the sounds you're hearing provide you with a negative or positive feeling. If you hear someone screaming at you, does it remind you of the past? Bring your attention back to the present moment. What's actually happening now?

Sometimes a loved one's anger might be directed at you, but it has nothing to do with how you're caring for him or her. Remember, the person in your care is also projecting what he or she is reflecting. You cannot control these reflections. If your loved one becomes upset, don't respond in anger. You can point out that what he or she is saying is inappropriate, or you can leave the room and come back when your loved one has more control over his or her behavior.

Reflect with smelling

Certain aromas can inspire you or relax you. The smell of fresh rainwater renews my spirit and gives me hope for the future. When I feel stressed out, I imagine it's raining and reflect back to the way the fresh water smells. You can try out some of the many aroma therapy products on the market, including oils and candles. On the go and don't have time for aroma therapy? Reflect back to your childhood and the smells of your favorite meal when you were growing up. I love to recall the smell of Mom's freshly baked chocolate chip cookies.

Reflect with touch

Touch allows us to feel and to experience the world. When I feel burned out, I often cuddle into a quilt my grandmother made for me when I was a young child. I also use the same blanket when I think I'm coming down with a cold. Something about touching this blanket renews my spirit. It reminds me of the unconditional love my grandmother had for me.

Reflect with tasting

Certain foods may bring back negative or positive thoughts and feelings. If you're feeling stressed, indulge in a sweet treat or eat a piece of fresh fruit. When I need to be nurtured, I like eating red Jell-o and macaroni and cheese. These foods remind me of my childhood, and I find them very comforting. What are some of your favorite foods? Don't let food start to control you, however. Too much of a good thing can interfere with healthy self-care.

The Benefits of Reflecting with Your Body

- Clarity about what is real versus perceived
- Reduction in anticipatory anxiety
- Freedom from the past
- Tranquility

Reflecting with Your Spirit

Reflecting with your spirit allows you to renew your body and mind. You can reflect with your spirit by learning to quiet your mind, silencing its inner chatter and images. Our minds seem to run nonstop with thoughts or images, and learning to silence your mind can be difficult, but with enough practice you'll succeed. As your mind becomes silent, you'll feel a refreshing sense of timelessness.

The silence in your mind and stillness in your body give you a chance to renew yourself and connect to your inner spirit. Before you had your thoughts or images, there was only silence. The genesis of all creation comes from this starting place of silence.

Many things can keep you from reflecting with your spirit, such as negative memories and worrying about the future, not to mention the daily demands of being a caregiver. It's easy to get so concerned about arranging transportation to medical appointments, making sure medications are taken on time, and finding the financial resources to cover the costs associated with caring for an ill person that your attention is mostly on past or future events rather than the present moment.

Worrying about things you cannot control or having feelings of regrets about the past can easily rob you of reflecting with your spirit. They can also lead to poor emotional and physical health. Learning to refrain from judging things as good or bad, right or wrong, will help you quiet your mind so that you can reflect with your spirit.

Remember how the elderly woman on a bike ride taught me the importance of focusing on one pedal at a time? I believe she had learned to reflect with her spirit and that knowledge gave her the strength and energy to do what others her age could not.

Success Story

Mona is a bank executive who shares in the responsibility of caring for her elderly mother with her younger brother. Mona's brother lives out of state but contributes financially to their mother's well-being. Mona appreciates the financial contribution but sometimes feels resentful because her brother is not in town to handle many of the daily caregiving duties.

Every Friday Mona takes her mother out for lunch and then to the store to buy groceries. One day while returning from the grocery store, Mona's mother fell in the hallway leading to her apartment. Mona had been under a lot of stress at work, and when her mother fell down, Mona also collapsed out of emotional and physical exhaustion.

The anticipation of additional care needs for Mona's mom was too much for her to handle, and Mona allowed her thoughts to gain control of her body, causing her to faint.

Mona became conscious before the paramedics arrived to care for her mother and took several deep breaths to help herself connect to the present moment.

When she realized what had happened, she began to reflect with her spirit, letting her mind be silent. This silence allowed her to gain control over her thoughts and body and she did not permit the anticipation of things that may or may not happen to her mother to affect her tranquility. Taking just a few moments to silence her mind and reflect with her spirit gave Mona the energy and focus to better care for her mother.

What You Can Do

Reflect in the moment

All you really have is the present moment. Becoming conscious of the present moment is the first step in reflecting with your spirit.

Reflect in silence

Learn to quiet your mind. Observe the conversation of your inner voice. As you learn to listen to your inner voice, you'll notice that behind it is an ever-present silence.

Reflect through acceptance

The voice we use to judge others is the same voice we use to judge ourselves. Refraining from external judgment will soon result in the absence of internal judgment.

Reflect by surrendering

Knowing that you don't have to have all the answers can be uplifting and can make it easier for you to be in touch with your spirit.

The Benefits of Reflecting with Your Spirit

- Reduction in depression and anxiety
- Living a life of authenticity
- Being present with others
- Experiencing the power to transform
- Sense of renewal

Concluding Thoughts on Reflecting

What you reflect on can determine how you feel, and negative reflections can cause caregiver burnout. With this knowledge you are able to make a positive change for yourself and your loved one. Learn to quiet your mind, silencing thoughts and images.

When you change what you reflect on and live in the present moment, you're turning wasted energy into renewable energy to care for yourself and your loved one.

You can renew yourself and ascend up the caregiving staircase by reflecting with your mind, body, and spirit. The more aligned your mind, body, and spirit are, the easier your caregiver ascent will be.

Conclusion

The sun had begun to set. The shadow of the Franklin Mountains was cascading over the border town of El Paso, Texas, a place I called home for the first thirty years of my life. It was Halloween night in 1984, and cars from across the border were cruising the streets of our middle-class neighborhood. From time to time, the cars would stop and idle as the young ghosts and goblins poured out into the streets scouring the neighborhood for sweets. The candy was collected in pillowcases, brown paper bags, and orange pumpkin-shaped buckets. The young ones ate some of the candy as they made their journey up and down our neighborhood streets. Most of it they took home to share with their younger brothers and sisters back in Juárez across the Rio Grande.

The tart breeze of the southwest desert and the innocence of youthful laughter entered my childhood home as my dad opened the front door to greet his visitors. Dad found joy in experiences that affirmed he was still valuable, and he fought hard for his independence despite the challenges of his poor health and advancing age. His skeletal frame was barely a reflection of the athletic build he once had. Chronic disease had taken over his physical body, leaving only the beauty of his spirit.

When Dad opened the door, the young children were startled by the image before them, and their laughter was silenced. Dad was dressed in a pair of flannel pajamas too large for his small frame. On the right side of his waist was a kidney dialysis bag that was connected to the center of his abdomen. Coach Watkins offered each one of the children a piece of candy from the candy dish Mom had set out earlier in the day. Being legally blind, he could no longer make the distinction, as each child came forward, between boy or girl, Anglo or Latino. He was munching on a piece of candy himself, though he couldn't chew it since his teeth have been missing for years.

The children stood in line quiet and mesmerized by the man they saw before them, as if they were experiencing communion for the very first time. Upon receiving the candy, each child stared gently at my dad before walking back to the curb.

After the children left, I began scolding Dad for opening the door without assistance. Dad shut the door and bowed his head with a sense of despair, and then I began a second round of verbal attacks at him for giving candy to kids who weren't from our own neighborhood. Gently, my dad turned to me with tears in his eyes and a smile. Humbly and with grace, he handed me the candy dish and said quietly, "We are all children of God."

It's been almost two decades since my father's death, but I still hear those words every time I feel disconnected from someone in my care. His words inspire me into action—to serve every child of God I can, regardless of our differences. They also remind me that the way we communicate makes all the difference in whether our caregiving experience is a satisfying one or not—for ourselves and those in our care.

The Halloween experience with my dad helped me see that what I was reflecting on and projecting was disconnecting me from him and others and eliminating my joy. So much of my focus had been on the illness and not on his strengths and on how to have a loving, supportive relationship with him. The way I was communicating was hurting my dad and burning me out. I'm grateful I have since learned the skills of CPR. It's now easier for me to find joy in being a caregiver and to renew myself when the going gets tough.

As you climb the caregiving spiral, becoming at risk for burnout, you can make positive changes for yourself and the people you care for by communicating through CPR. Start using CPR today. You'll become your own renewable resource and experience the joy in caregiving.

About the Author

Grant Watkins began his twenty-plus years of caregiving at the age of seventeen, when his father was declared legally blind. For more than five years, Grant experienced caregiver fatigue while sharing the responsibilities of caring for his father, who died shortly after his twenty-second birthday. Despite the heavy burden and fatigue, the experience of caring for his father also allowed Grant to feel powerful moments of intense love that transformed his life.

Grant founded Mission for Mobility in 2002 as a community service initiative in which he now serves as an inspirational speaker. In addition to inspiring caregivers, he strives to empower people to live independently.

Grant, who holds a bachelor of arts in communications, currently works for a nonprofit organization that promotes independent living for seniors and for those who have chronic physical and/or mental disabilities.